Mediterranean Diet Recipes Book

Improve Your Diet & Lifestyle With These 50 Mediter ranean Delicous Dishes

Carlo Montesanti

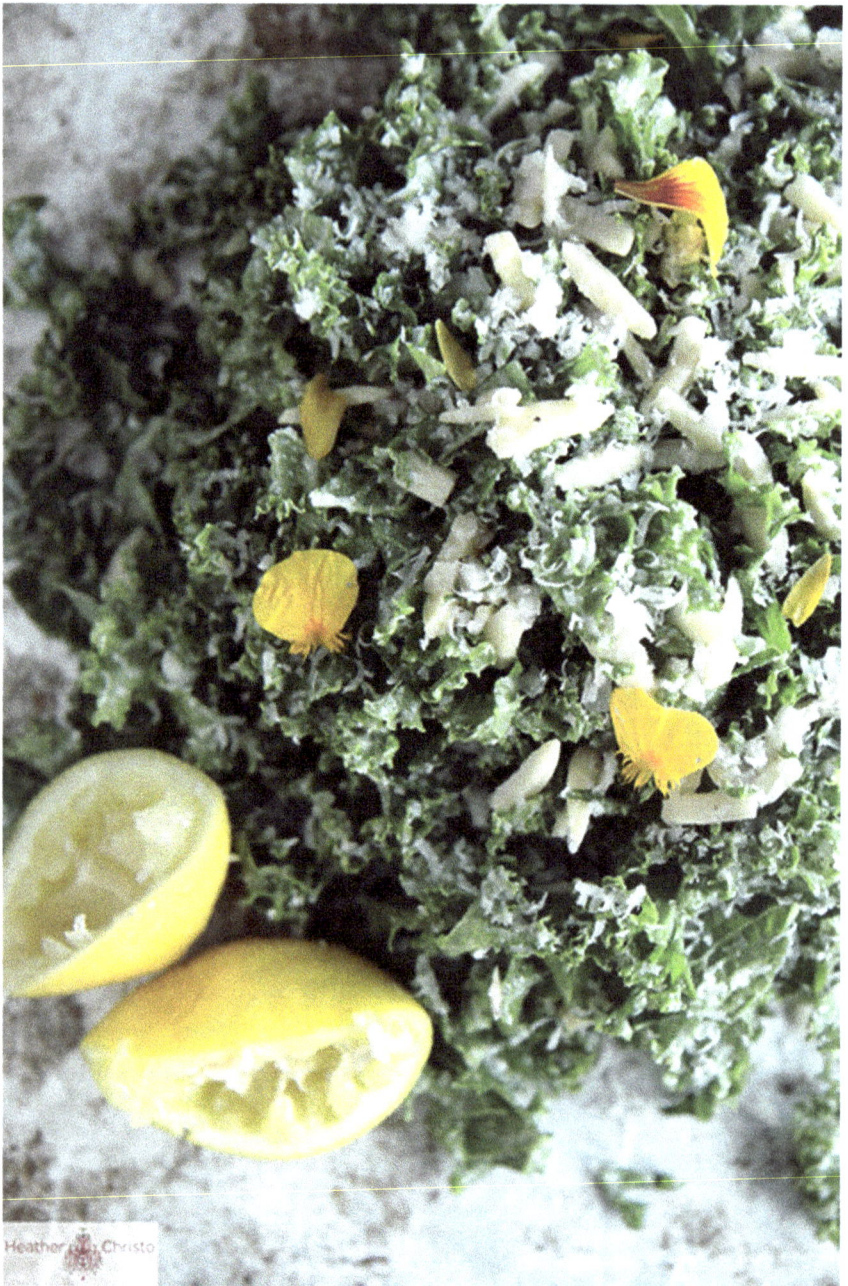

Table of Contents

Kale Salad with Pecorino and Lemon

Prep Time: 5 min

Cook Time: 0 min

Serve: 4

Ingredients:

- 1 large bunch kale, washed and trimmed of steams

- lemons, juiced

- ounces Pecorino Romano, grated

- ½ cup olive oil

- Kosher salt and fresh black pepper to taste

Preparation:

1. Wrap several cabbage leaves lengthwise and cut off the thick central stem using the tip of a knife. On the other hand, wrap the remaining pile of dehydrated leaves in a tight cigar shape and cut them into thin ribbons.

2. Discard the grated cabbage with the cheese. Lightly beat the lemon juice and olive oil and pour over the salad. Try and season with salt and pepper. Let the salad sit at room temperature for an hour before serving.

Venison Tenderloin

Prep Time: 20 min

Cook Time: 75 min

Serve: 6

Ingredients:

- 4 pounds venison tenderloin

- 2 sprigs fresh thyme

- 2 sprigs fresh rosemary

- Two cloves garlic, crushed

- Two bay leaves

- One medium onion, chopped

- 1 cup red wine

- ½ cup apple cider vinegar

Preparation:

1. Add red wine cider vinegar, garlic, bay leaves, thyme, rosemary & onion in a cup & blend them. Move it to the large jar, & place in the bag the venison tenderloin.

2. Close it tightly, and make it airtight. Then place the meat in a refrigerator for marination for at least 13 hours, turn it 2 or 3 times. Preheated the oven to 325°F (165 °C).

3. Take Off meat away from the marinade & put it in a roasting rack. Roast it for two to two and a half hours in the oven. The Internal roasting temperature would be a minimum of 150 °F.

4. Let the roast rest for 10 to 15 minutes before cutting.

5. Heat the sauce over low heat in a pan as the side roasts.

6. Boil till there is a 1/3 drop in the oil. Serve & Enjoy.

Seared venison with plum ginger sauce and vermicelli sauce

Prep Time: 10 min

Cook Time: 15 min

Serve: 2

Ingredients:

- Vermicelli salad
- One carrot grated
- One red capsicum sliced
- 100 g snow peas sliced
- 100 g vermicelli noodles
- Two tbsp Thai basil leaves chopped
- Venison and plum sauce
- ¼ cup red wine

- One clove garlic minced

- One tablespoon soy sauce

- One teaspoon ginger finely grated

- Two tablespoons plum jam

- 300 g venison medallions

Dressing:

- ½ teaspoon sesame oil

- One tablespoon olive oil

- One tablespoon soy sauce

- One teaspoon plum jam

- One tablespoon Thai basil leaves chopped

- One tablespoon sesame seeds

Preparation:

1. Bring to the boil a full pot.

2. Use a Proof heat Bowl, place the vermicelli noodles in the bowl and pour over the boiling water to cover them. Threads are detached by stirring, covering with a plate, and leaving until smooth, around 4 minutes. Threads are

shortened by cutting the threads from different places using kitchen scissors. Apply oil in a small amount to avoid Sticking.

3. Use paper towels, Dry the venison, and season it with salt. 4. Heat the saucepan to medium temperature. Toast sesame seeds until crispy and fragrant for 1 to 2 minutes. Add a drizzle of oil and raise the heat. Once cooked, grill the venison for 2 to 3 minutes on both sides. Cover the venison with foil.

5. Return the pan to low heat for the plum sauce and apply a small amount of oil. Fry the ginger and garlic for 30 seconds, stir-fry the red wine, and boil until halved. Now add plum jelly, fresh plums, and soy sauce and boil until slightly thickened, and stir for around 1 minute. Use black pepper for seasoning. If the sauce gets too thick and jam-like, give a splash of water to thin it out to a decent pouring consistency. Stir in the sleeping venison juices.

6. Mix all of the ingredients in a big dish. Add all the salad ingredients leftover, the noodles, and toss to coat. Season with salt and pepper.

7. Divide the vermicelli salad between the plates to serve. Cover with venison and drizzle all over the sauce with plum.

8. Sprinkle the Thai basil and sesame seeds.

Venison Stir-Fry

Prep Time: 20 min

Cook Time: 5 min

Serve: 4

Ingredients:

Marinade

- 1/2 teaspoon salt

- Two tablespoons

- Shaoxing wine or dry sherry

- Three tablespoons soy sauce

- One tablespoon potato starch Stir fry

- 1 1/2 cups peanut or other cooking oil

- 1 pound venison, trimmed of fat

- 1 to 4 fresh red chiles

- One red or yellow bell pepper, sliced

- Three garlic cloves, slivered

- One bunch cilantro, roughly chopped

- One tablespoon soy sauce

- Two teaspoons sesame oil

Preparation:

1. Cut the venison into small slivers between 1/4 inch or less and 1 to 3 inches in length from anywhere. Mix and set aside with the marinade as you cut out all the remaining ingredients.

2. Heat a big heavy pot with the peanut oil until it reaches 275 °F to 290°F. Apply about 1/3 of venison to hot oil and use a chopstick or a butter knife to separate the meat slices.

3. Let them sizzle for 30 - 60 seconds. Set aside and cook one-third at a time for the remaining venison.

4. Pour all but only three tablespoons of the oil out of it.

5. Keep the remaining oil hot. Add up the chiles and the bell peppers. Stir-fry for 90 seconds when it starts to burn, add garlic, and cook for an extra 30 seconds. Add the venison and fry for 90 seconds and stir.

6. Add the coriander and soy sauce and fry for the remaining 30 seconds before the coriander wilts. Turn the heat off, then whisk in the sesame oil. Serve with steamed rice at once.

Lamb, apricot & shallot tagine

Prep Time: 30 min

Cook Time: 7 h 30 min

Serve: 5-6

Ingredients:

- 1 tbsp clear honey

- 1 tbsp ras el hanout

- One large leg of lamb, bone-in (about 2kg)

- 150ml hot chicken stock

- Two preserved lemons

- 400g small apricot, halved and stoned

- 600g shallot, halved if particularly large

- 85g whole skinless almond

- couscous and natural yogurt, to serve little pack coriander leaves picked

For the marinade

- 1 tbsp ground cumin

- 2 tbsp clear honey

- 1 tsp coriander seed

- 2 tsp ground cinnamon

- 2 tsp ground ginger

- 4 tbsp olive oil

- Four garlic cloves, crushed pinch of saffron strands

Preparation:

1. Cut the lamb's leg all over and put it in a large bag of food. 2. Using the pestle and mortar, shatter the marinade ingredients simultaneously. Brush over the entire lamb with black pepper. Overnight, or up to 24 hours, to marinate.

3. Place the lamb in a large roasting tin, removing any residual marinade from the top. Use foil to protect the container, and close the foil from the ends. Cook for 6-7 hours, basting until the beef is extremely tender.

4. Drop the oven roasting tin and raise the oven to 200°C /180°C. Pour into a measuring jug the juices from the

lamb, slightly cool it, and remove the fat off. Place the shallots with the lamb in the tin and toss in some of the juices to coat them. Roast the apricots and almonds for 15 mins, and then add them. Whisk the lemon, honey, ras el hanout, and stock in the cooking juices, then pour on the lamb and then roast again for 20 mins.

5. Leave it for 10 minutes, then scatter and eat with couscous and yogurt over the herbs.

Flank Steak, Broccoli and Green Bean Stir-Fry

Prep Time: 15 min

Cook Time: 12 min

Ingredients:

- 3 cups cooked brown rice

- Two tablespoons vegetable oil

- Two tablespoons rice vinegar

- One ¼ pound lean beef flank steak

- 1 cup beef broth

- One tablespoon cornstarch

- One head broccoli, cut into florets (about 6 cups)

- 1 cup shredded carrot

- ½ teaspoon red pepper flakes

- ½ teaspoon Chinese five-spice powder

- ½ pound thin green beans, trimmed

- ½ large onion, sliced

- ½ cup sliced almonds

- ¼ teaspoon salt

- ¼ cup reduced-sodium soy sauce

Preparation:

1. Combine the soy sauce, broth, 5-spice powder, vinegar, cornstarch, & the red chili flakes in a cup and place it aside.

2. Take a non-stick fry pan, add 1 tbsp of oil to it, and heat it. Pepper the salted stir-fry flank steak & for 4 minutes. Remove to a tray. Add the remaining one tbsp. Of oil in it, and then add broccoli, cabbage, green beans, & carrot. Stir-cook for 9 minutes or till it becomes soft & crisp.

3. Add ¼ cup of water at the last two minutes of cooking time. Now add a mixture of soya sauce& broth in it and then boil & simmer it for 2 minutes, until well dense. Stir in some stored juices & beef & heat up. Decorate with the almonds & serve with the cooked brown rice instantly.

Moroccan beef tagine

Prep Time: 25 min

Cook Time: 7 hrs

Serve: 4

Ingredients:

Marinade

- pinch of sea salt
- pinch of ground cardamon
- 1 tsp ground sweet paprika
- 1 tsp ground ginger
- 1 tsp ground cumin
- 1 tsp ground cinnamon
- 1 tsp dried rose petals
- 1 tbsp ras el hanout
- 1 tbsp olive oil

Tagine

- One onion, peeled and chopped

- 1 tbsp olive oil for frying

- 400 g of chickpeas

- 400 g chopped tomatoes

- 150 g prunes, sliced

- 150 ml of beef stock

- Two carrots sliced

- Four small tomatoes quartered

- 400 g butternut squash, diced

- 600 g diced stewing beef

- fresh coriander

Preparation:

1. Combine all marinade items in a small glass.

2. Take a dish, place beef in it, pour marinade all over it & mix it well for coating all-beef parts equally.

3. Cover bowl with foil & refrigerate it for 3 to 4 hours.

4. Take a frying pan, add oil in it, heat it, add onions and fry for 3 to 4 minutes, then add beef in it and fry it for 5 to 6 minutes until it turned brown.

5. In a boiled slow oven dish, pass by the onion & beef.

6. Add & stock the tinned tomatoes along with onions, quartered tomatoes &, stir well, add the onions, quartered tomatoes, & butternut squash, & then mix again.

7. Turn on the auto mode, cover a slow cooker, & keep a dish simmer for 7 to 8 hours until the beef is very tender. Add the prunes & chickpeas for one hour till cooking ends. Serve with splattered couscous with finely sliced coriander.

Persian Roast Lamb

Prep Time: 20 min

Cook Time: 150 min

Serve: 8

Ingredients:

- One large onion sliced or chopped
- 1 tbsp EV olive oil
- 1 tbsp ground cumin
- tsp ground black pepper
- 1 tsp turmeric
- One leg or shoulder of lamb
- Two strips of fresh rosemary
- 2 Tbsp honey
- Tbsp liquid saffron
- 250 ml of vegetable stock
- 4 tbsp pomegranate molasses

- Five cloves garlic finely chopped or crushed

- One lemon juice

- Marinade

Preparation:

1. Preheat micro to 180 deg C. Make slashes. Mix ingredients & rub them over the lamb.

2. Line sliced onions with a preferred dish. Pour the stock.

3. Remember to Pour on onions. Cover using foil & roast for 60 minutes. Have the lamb wrapped in aluminum foil with a wonderful sauce.

Stir-fried garlic chili beef and ong Choi

Prep Time: 8 min

Cook Time: 15 min

Serve: 2

Ingredients:

- 200g beef fillet, sliced into even-sized thin strips

- Few pinches Chinese five-spice

- Light soy sauce to season

- 1 tbsp groundnut oil

- Four large garlic cloves, finely chopped

- 150 ong Choi, washed, leaves and stems cut across the stem in equal 10cm lengths (or use spinach or watercress)

- One medium red chili, de-seeded and finely chopped Toasted sesame oil, to season

Preparation:

1. Season the beef with soy sauce. Toss well. Heat a saucepan. Add oil & garlic. Fry 30 sec. Add beef & stir.

2. Apply one Choi & chili. Season with light soy sauce, sea salt, & sesame oil splashes for serving.

3. Serve immediately & enjoy.

Asian Broccoli and Ginger Salad

Prep Time: 10 min

Cook Time: 10 min

Serve: 4

Ingredients:

- Salt and pepper to taste

- Three tablespoons low sodium soy sauce

- Three tablespoons balsamic vinegar

- Two cloves garlic minced

- Two teaspoons brown sugar

- 2 cups sugar snap peas

- 1/4 cup almonds

- One red pepper julienne cut

- 1 (12 ounces) bag broccoli coleslaw

- One tablespoon fresh ginger

- 1 1/2 teaspoons sesame oil

Preparation:

1. Mix soy sauce, garlic, sesame oil, vinegar, brown sugar, & ginger. Put it aside for a while. Steam sugar snaps for roughly 3-4 min.

2. For stopping the cooking process, immerse it in an ice bath. Drain well. Mix peas, almonds, broccoli coleslaw, red pepper & sesame ginger. Dressing in a big dish.

3. Add salt to taste & black pepper powder.

Avocado and three-bean salad

Prep Time: 15 min

Cook Time: 15 min

Serve: 8

Ingredients:

- salt and pepper to taste

- juice of 2 limes

- Two large avocados, peeled, pitted, and diced

- Two cloves garlic, mashed or finely diced

- 12 grape or cherry tomatoes, halved

- 1/3 cup olive oil

- One large orange or red bell pepper, diced

- One bunch cilantro, chopped

- 15 oz kernel corn

- 15 oz red kidney beans

- 15 oz garbanzo beans

- 15 oz black beans

Preparation:

1. Take a big bowl. Combine all ingredients. Refrigerate for 60 minutes before serving.

2. Tossed it with lime. Serve & enjoy.

Baked Adzuki Beans with Aubergine & Tomatoes

Prep time: 8 min

Cook time: 90 min

Serve: 6

Ingredients:

- One bouquet garni (thyme, parsley, and bay leaf)

- cup chicken stock (or one bouillon cube dissolved in 1 cup water)

- 1 cup dried adzuki beans

- One onion, finely chopped

- ½ cup fresh grated parmesan cheese

- ½ teaspoon ground allspice

- ¼ teaspoon red pepper flakes

- Two cloves garlic, minced

- Two sliced eggplants

- ½ cups canned chopped tomatoes

- Four tablespoons fresh basil, shredded

- Six tablespoons olive oil

- kosher salt or sea salt

- salt and pepper, to taste

Preparation:

1. Add garlic & boil water. Reduce heat & simmer before beans become soft for 50 minutes. Preheat microwave to 375°. Heat olive oil in a frying pan on moderate heat.

2. Move to bake dish. Heat leftover olive oil pan & sauté onion before it begins to soften.

3. Add garlic & sauté for one min. Add tomatoes, red pepper flakes, salt, allspice, & black pepper. Blend well.

4. Sprinkle with cheese & bake for 20 min. Serve & enjoy.

Roasted Sorghum

Prep Time: 10 min

Cook Time: 15 min

Serve: 4

Ingredients:

- tbsp. avocado oil

- ½ cup sorghum, cooked

- 1 carrot, diced

- tbsp. dried parsley

- ½ tsp. dried oregano

- 2 tbsp. cream cheese

Preparation:

1. Heat avocado oil and add the carrot. Roast it for 5 minutes. Then add cooked sorghum, parsley, oregano, and cream cheese.

2. Roast the meal for 10 minutes on low heat. Stir it from time to time to avoid burning.

Sorghum Stew

Prep Time: 10 min

Cook Time: 25 min

Serve: 5

Ingredients:

- 1 cup sorghum
- ½ cup ground sausages
- ½ cup tomatoes
- 1 jalapeno pepper, chopped
- ½ cup bell pepper, chopped
- 4 cups chicken stock

Preparation:

1. Roast the sausages for 5 minutes in the saucepan. Then add tomatoes, jalapeno, and bell pepper.

Cook the ingredients for 10 minutes.

2. After this, add sorghum and chicken stock and boil the stew for 10 minutes more.

Sorghum Salad

Prep Time: 10 min

Cook Time: 10 min

Serve: 3

Ingredients:

- 3 oz butternut squash, chopped

- ¼ cup sorghum

- ¼ cup fresh cilantro, chopped

- 1 tsp. ground cumin

- cups water

- 2 tbsp. organic canola oil

- 2 tbsp. apple cider vinegar

Preparation:

1. Put sorghum and butternut squash in the saucepan. Add water and cook for 10 minutes. Then cool the ingredients and transfer in the salad bowl.

2. Add cilantro, ground cumin, organic canola oil, and apple cider vinegar. Stir the meal well.

Sorghum Bake

Prep Time: 10 min

Cook Time: 25 min

Serve: 4

Ingredients:

- ½ cup sorghum

- 1 apple, chopped

- 1 oz raisins

- 1.5cup of water

Preparation:

1. Put sorghum in the pan. Flatten it. Then top it with raisins, apple, and water. Cover the meal with baking paper and transfer in the preheated to 375F oven.

2. Bake the meal for 25 minutes.

Lamb and Chickpeas Stew

Prep Time: 10 min

Cook Time: 1 h 20 min

Serve: 6

Ingredients:

- 1 and ½ lb. lamb shoulder, cubed

- 3 tbsp. olive oil

- 1 cup yellow onion, chopped

- 1 cup carrots, cubed

- 1 cup celery, chopped

- 3 garlic cloves, minced

- 4 rosemary springs, chopped

- 2 cups chicken stock

- 1 cup tomato puree

- 15 oz. canned chickpeas, drained and rinsed

- 10 oz. baby spinach

- 2 tbsp. black olives, pitted and sliced

- A pinch of salt and black pepper

Preparation:

1. Heat a pot with the oil over medium-high heat, add the meat, salt and pepper and brown for 5 minutes.

2. Add carrots, celery, onion and garlic, stir and sauté for 5 minutes more. Add the rosemary, stock, chickpeas and the other ingredients except the spinach and olives, stir and cook for 1 hour.

3. Add the rest of the ingredients, cook the stew over medium heat for 10 minutes more, divide into bowls and serve.

Chorizo and Lentils Stew

Prep Time: 10 min

Cook Time: 35 min

Serve: 4

Ingredients:

- 4 cups water

- 1 cup carrots, sliced

- 1 yellow onion, chopped

- 1 tbsp. extra-virgin olive oil

- ¾ cup celery, chopped

- 1 and ½ tsp. garlic, minced

- 1 and ½ lb. gold potatoes, roughly chopped

- 7 oz. chorizo, cut in half lengthwise and thinly sliced

- 1 and ½ cup lentils

- ½ tsp. smoked paprika

- ½ tsp. oregano

- Salt and black pepper to taste

- 14 oz. canned tomatoes, chopped

- ½ cup cilantro, chopped

Preparation:

1. Heat a saucepan with oil over medium high heat, add onion, garlic, celery and carrots, stir and cook for 4 minutes.

2. Add the chorizo, stir and cook for 1 minute more.

3. Add the rest of the ingredients except the cilantro, stir, bring to a boil, reduce heat to medium-low and simmer for 25 minutes. Divide the stew into bowls and serve with the cilantro sprinkled on top. Enjoy!

Lamb and Potato Stew

Prep Time: 10 min

Cook Time: 2 h

Serve: 4

Ingredients:

- 2 and ½ lb. lamb shoulder, boneless and cut in small pieces Salt and black pepper to taste
- 1 yellow onion, chopped
- 3 tbsp. extra virgin olive oil
- 3 tomatoes, grated
- and ½ cups chicken stock
- ½ cup dry white wine
- 1 bay leaf
- ½ lb. gold potatoes, cut into medium cubes
- ¾ cup green olives

Preparation:

1. Heat a saucepan with the oil over medium high heat, add the lamb, brown for 10 minutes, transfer to a platter and keep warm for now. Heat the pan again, add onion, stir and cook for 4 minutes. Add tomatoes, stir, reduce heat to low and cook for 15 minutes.

2. Return lamb meat to pan, add wine and the rest of the ingredients except the potatoes and olives, stir, increase heat to medium high, bring to a boil, reduce heat again, cover pan and simmer for 30 minutes.

3. Add potatoes and olives, stir, cook for 1 more hour, divide into bowls and serve.

Meatball and Pasta Soup

Prep Time: 10 min

Cook Time: 40 min

Serve: 4

Ingredients:

- 12 oz. pork meat, ground

- 12 oz. veal, ground

- Salt and black pepper to taste

- 1 garlic clove, minced

- garlic cloves, sliced

- 2 tsp. thyme, chopped

- 1 egg, whisked

- oz. Manchego, grated

- 2 tbsp. extra virgin olive oil

- 1/3 cup panko

- 4 cups chicken stock

- A pinch of saffron

- 15 oz. canned tomatoes, crushed

- 1 tbsp. parsley, chopped

- 8 oz. pasta

Preparation:

1. In a bowl, mix veal with pork, 1 garlic clove, 1 tsp. thyme, ¼ tsp. paprika, salt, pepper to taste, egg, manchego, panko, stir very well and shape medium meatballs out of this mix.

2. Heat a pan with 1 ½ tbsp. oil over medium high heat, add half of the meatballs, cook for 2 minutes on each side, transfer to paper towels, drain grease and put on a plate.

3. Repeat this with the rest of the meatballs.

4. Heat a saucepan with the rest of the oil, add sliced garlic, stir and cook for 1 minute.

5. Add the remaining ingredients and the meatballs, stir, reduce heat to medium low, cook for 25 minutes and season with salt and pepper. Cook pasta according to instructions, drain, put in a bowl and mix with ½ cup soup.

6. Divide pasta into soup bowls, add soup and meatballs on top, sprinkle parsley all over and serve.

Peas Soup

Prep Time: 10 min

Cook Time: 10 min

Serve: 4

Ingredients:

- 1 tsp. shallot, chopped

- 1 tbsp. butter

- quart chicken stock

- 2 eggs

- 3 tbsp. lemon juice

- 2 cups peas

- tbsp. parmesan, grated

- Salt and black pepper to taste

Preparation:

1. Heat a saucepan with the butter over medium high heat, add shallot, stir and cook for 2 minutes.

2. Add stock, lemon juice, some salt and pepper and the whisked eggs.

3. Add more salt and pepper to taste, peas and parmesan cheese, stir, cook for 3 minutes, divide into bowls and serve.

Minty Lamb Stew

Prep Time: 10 min

Cook Time: 1 h 45 min

Serve: 4

Ingredients:

- cups orange juice

- ½ cup mint tea

- Salt and black pepper to taste

- 2 lb. lamb shoulder chops

- 1 tbsp. mustard, dry

- 3 tbsp. canola oil

- 1 tbsp. ras el hanout

- 1 carrot, chopped

- 1 yellow onion, chopped

- 1 celery rib, chopped

- 1 tbsp. ginger, grated

- 28 oz. canned tomatoes, crushed

- 1 tbsp. garlic, minced

- star anise

- 1 cup apricots, dried and cut in halves

- 1 cinnamon stick

- ½ cup mint, chopped

- 15 oz. canned chickpeas, drained

- 6 tbsp. yogurt

Preparation:

1. Put orange juice in a saucepan, bring to a boil over medium heat, take off heat, add tea leaves, cover and leave aside for 3 minutes, strain this and leave aside.

2. Heat a saucepan with 2 tbsp. oil over medium high heat, add lamb chops seasoned with salt, pepper, mustard and rasel hanout, toss, brown for 3 minutes on each side and transfer to a plate. Add remaining oil to the saucepan, heat over medium heat, add ginger, onion, carrot, garlic and celery, stir and cook for 5 minutes.

3. Add orange juice, star anise, tomatoes, cinnamon stick, lamb, apricots, stir and cook for 1 hour and 30 minutes.

4. Transfer lamb chops to a cutting board, discard bones and chop. Bring sauce from the pan to a boil, add chickpeas and mint, stir and cook for 10 minutes.

5. Discard cinnamon and star anise, divide into bowls and serve with yogurt on top.

Spinach and Orzo Soup

Prep Time: 10 min

Cook Time: 10 min

Serve: 4

Ingredients:

- ½ cup orzo

- 6 cups chicken soup

- and ½ cups parmesan, grated

- Salt and black pepper to taste

- 1 and ½ tsp. oregano, dried

- ¼ cup yellow onion, finely chopped

- 3 cups baby spinach

- tbsp. lemon juice

- ½ cup peas, frozen

Preparation:

1. Heat a saucepan with the stock over high heat, add oregano, orzo, onion, salt and pepper, stir, bring to a boil, cover and cook for 10 minutes.

2. Take soup off the heat, add salt and pepper to taste and the rest of the ingredients, stir well and divide into soup bowls. Serve right away.

Minty Lentil and Spinach Soup

Prep Time: 10 min

Cook Time: 30 min

Serve: 6

Ingredients:

- 2 tbsp. olive oil

- 1 yellow onion, chopped

- A pinch of salt and black pepper

- 2 garlic cloves, minced

- 1 tsp. coriander, ground

- 1 tsp. cumin, ground

- 1 tsp. sumac

- 1 tsp. red pepper, crushed

- 2 tsp. mint, dried

- 1 tbsp. flour

- 6 cups veggie stock

- 3 cups water

- 12 oz. spinach, torn

- 1 and ½ cups brown lentils, rinsed

- 2 cups parsley, chopped

- Juice of 1 lime

Preparation:

1. Heat a pot with the oil over medium heat, add the onions, stir and sauté for 5 minutes.

2. Add garlic, salt, pepper, coriander, cumin, sumac, red pepper, mint and flour, stir and cook for another minute.

3.. Add the stock, water and the other ingredients except the parsley and lime juice, stir, bring to a simmer and cook for 20 minutes. Add the parsley and lime juice, cook the soup for 5 minutes more, ladle into bowls and serve.

Chicken and Apricots Stew

Prep Time: 10 min

Cook Time: 2 h 10 min

Serve: 4

Ingredients:

- 3 garlic cloves, minced

- 1 tbsp. parsley, chopped

- 20 saffron threads

- 3 tbsp. cilantro, chopped

- Salt and black pepper to taste

- 1 tsp. ginger, ground

- tbsp. olive oil

- red onions, thinly sliced

- 4 chicken drumsticks

- 5 oz. apricots, dried

- 2 tbsp. butter

- ¼ cup honey

- 2/3 cup walnuts, chopped

- ½ cinnamon stick

Preparation:

1. Heat a pan over medium high heat, add saffron threads, toast them for 2 minutes, transfer to a bowl, cool down and crush. Add the chicken pieces, 1 tbsp. cilantro, parsley, garlic, ginger, salt, pepper, oil and 2 tbsp. water, toss well and keep in the fridge for 30 minutes.

2. Arrange onion on the bottom of a saucepan.

3. Add chicken and marinade, add 1 tbsp. butter, place on stove over medium high heat and cook for 15 minutes.

4. Add ¼ cup water, stir, cover pan, reduce heat to medium- low and simmer for 45 minutes.

5. Heat a pan over medium heat, add 2 tbsp. honey, cinnamon stick, apricots and ¾ cup water, stir, bring to a boil, reduce to low and simmer for 15 minutes.

6. Take off heat, discard cinnamon and leave to cool down.

7. Heat a pan with remaining butter over medium heat, add remaining honey and walnuts, stir, cook for 5 minutes and transfer to a plate. Add chicken to apricot sauce, also season with salt, pepper and the rest of the cilantro stir, cook for 10 minutes and serve on top of walnuts.

Scallops and Summer

Vegetable Skillet

Prep Time: 15 min

Cook Time: 15 min

Serve: Adjustable

Ingredients:

- 1/2 cup diced zucchini

- 1 cup corn kernels

- One sliced cherry tomatoes

- 1 lb scallops

- 1 tbsp olive oil

- Three cloves garlic minced

- 3 tbsp diced shallots

- 3 tbsp salted butter

- Salt to taste pepper to taste

Preparation:

1. Cook scallops in a heated oven over medium flame for three minutes. Transfer it to a plate. Sauté shallots and garlic in the same pan over medium flame. Stir in zucchini and tomatoes for ten minutes.

2. Mix in corn, salt, and black pepper. Add scallop and cook for five minutes.

Tuna Patties

Prep Time: 15 min

Cook Time: 10 min

Serve: 4

Ingredients:

- 3 tbsp vegetable oil

- 3 tbsp grated Parmesan cheese

- 3 tbsp diced Onion

- 15 oz tuna

- 2 tsp lemon juice

- Two eggs

- 10 tbsp bread crumbs

- One pinch of black pepper

Preparation:

Whisk all the items in a bowl. Make patties out of the mixture. Fry the patties in heated oil over medium flame for five minutes.

Whole Salmon Fillet with Crispy Lemon & Basil Crumb Topping

Prep Time: 15 min

Cook Time: 18 min

Serve: 4

Ingredients:

- Salt to taste

- black pepper to taste

- Two cloves garlic

- 1.45 lb salmon fillet

- 1 tbsp lemon juice

- 1 tbsp lemon thyme

- 1 lb asparagus

- One lemon, zested

- 1 cup bread crumbs

- ½ tsp salt

- ½ tsp black pepper

- 1/3 cup grated Parmesan cheese

- 1/3 cup chopped fresh basil

- ¼ cup olive oil, divided

Preparation:

1. Season salmon with oil, pepper, and salt. Shift the salmon in the pan. Mix asparagus with oil and salt and place around salmon. Blend garlic, cheese, basil, thyme, lemon juice, zest, salt, and pepper in a food processor.

2. Pour the mixture over salmon. Bake in the oven for 20 minutes.

Seafood paella

Prep Time: 15 min

Cook Time: 55 min

Serve: 6

Ingredients:

- Two ¼ cups chicken broth

- 2 tsp olive oil

- 1 lb jumbo shrimp

- ½ teaspoon saffron threads

- salt to taste

- 8 oz sliced chorizo sausage

- Two cloves garlic, minced

- 1 1/3 cups Arborio rice

- 1 tsp paprika

- 1 tbsp olive oil

- One sliced red bell pepper

- One pinch of cayenne pepper

- ½ yellow onion, diced

- ½ cup green peas

Preparation:

1. Fry chorizo in heated oil for three minutes. Mix in onions and cook for three more minutes.

2. Stir in rice and peas and toss well. Place shrimp over rice and bake for twenty minutes.

Thyme-Scented Salmon with White Bean Salad

Prep Time: 15 min

Cook Time: 0 min

Serve: 4

Ingredients:

- Bean Salad

- 3 tbsp lemon juice

- 2 tsp chopped parsley

- 2 tsp chopped mint

- 2 tsp chopped basil

- 2 tbsp water

- Two garlic cloves, minced

- 1 tbsp olive oil

- 15 oz cannellini beans

- ½ cup chopped shallots

- ½ cup chopped carrot

- 1/3 cup chopped celery

- Salmon

- Four salmon fillets

- 3 tbsp lemon juice

- 2 tsp chopped thyme

- 13 tsp black pepper

- 1 tsp chopped parsley

- ½ tsp salt

Preparation:

1. Cook celery, carrot, shallots, and garlic in heated oil over medium flame for five minutes. Mix all the ingredients and cook. Place the mixture in salmon.

2. Bake salmon in a preheated oven at 375 degrees for 15 minutes.

Curry Chicken Salad

Prep Time: 15 min

Cook Time: 15 min

Serve: 6

Ingredients:

- Three cooked chicken breasts

- 2/3 cup chopped celery

- 2 tbsp lemon juice

- 1/4 tsp black pepper

- 1/4 cup sliced chives

- 1/3 cup raisins

- 1/2 tsp salt

- 1/2 cup roasted salted cashews

- 1/2 cup mayonnaise

- 1 tbsp yellow curry powder

- One tart apple

Preparation:

Whisk all the items in the bowl and serve.

Grilled Indian Chicken

Prep Time: 35 min

Cook Time: 10 min

Serve: 4

Ingredients:

- 4 boneless chicken breasts

Marinade

- 1/4 tsp cayenne pepper

- 1/2 tsp ginger

- 1/2 cup plain yogurt

- 1 tsp cumin

- 1 tsp coriander

- 1 tbsp paprika

- 1 tbsp onion powder

- 1 tbsp minced garlic

- 1 tbsp lemon juice

- 1 tbsp garam masala

- 1 tbsp cilantro leaves

Preparation:

Combine all the items in a bowl and set aside. Grill chicken over a grill for seven minutes from both sides.

Hearty Turkey Stew

Prep Time: 10 min

Cook Time: 60 min

Serve: 4

Ingredients:

- 100 g sliced bacon lardons

- 1/3 cup heavy cream

- 1 tbsp butter

- One leek

- Two sliced carrots

- Two stalks celery diced

- Two cloves garlic pressed

- 2 tbsp flour, heaped

- 4 cups chicken or turkey stock

- 2 cups cooked turkey

- Two chopped potatoes

- Two bay leaves

- 1 tbsp thyme leaves

- 1 tbsp chopped parsley

- salt to taste

- pepper to taste

Preparation:

1. Fry bacon in butter over medium flame. Stir in leeks, carrots, thyme, and celery, and cook for five minutes. Mix garlic and cook again for one minute.

2. Add flour, pepper, and salt. Mix potatoes, bay leaves, and turkey and cook for 50 minutes. Add heavy cream and serve.

Herb and Orange Chicken

Prep Time: 10 min

Cook Time: 60 min

Serve: 4

Ingredients:

- 1/4 cup ghee

- 3 1/2 oranges

- 4.5 lb chicken

- Three yellow potatoes

- Two stems of rosemary

- Six stems of thyme

- salt & pepper

Preparation:

Heat orange juice in ghee over medium flame and set aside.

Place chicken, potatoes, orange slices, thyme, and rosemary. Bake for one hour and serve with orange sauce.

Pomegranate Walnut & Chicken Stew

Prep Time: 15 min

Cook Time: 75 min

Serve: 5

Ingredients:

- 1 cups California walnuts

- pinch salt

- pepper

- 2 tbsp olive oil

- 1 tbsp butter

- Four cloves garlic chopped

- 1 tsp turmeric

- 1 tsp cumin

- One cinnamon stick

- ½ tsp nutmeg

- ½ tsp black pepper orange zest

- 2 cups chicken stock

- 2 tbsp maple

- 1 ½ tsp salt One chickpea

- serve with Persian Rice

- Garnish using chopped Italian parsley

- Garnish with pomegranate seeds

- 1–1 ½ lb chicken thighs

- 3 cups yellow onion, diced

- 1/4 cup pomegranate molasses

Preparation:

1. Roast the walnuts over medium flame. Blend the roasted walnuts. Cook chicken in a Dutch oven in heated oil. Set aside. Fry onions in heated oil for five minutes.

2. Stir in garlic and sauté for five minutes. Mix cinnamon, nutmeg, cumin, zest, and turmeric and sauté for a minute.

3. Pour in stock, chicken, syrup, molasses, walnuts, salt, and simmer for 45 minutes. Add the chickpeas and boil it for 15 minutes.

Roasted Chicken and White Bean Medley

Prep Time: 20 min

Cook Time: 60 min

Serve: 4

Ingredients:

- Eight teaspoons Dijon mustard

- Eight skin-on bone-in chicken thighs (about 2 pounds)

- Two tablespoons olive oil

- Two tablespoons coarsely chopped fresh parsley

- Two tablespoons capers with brine

- 2 (15-ounce) cans white beans, drained and rinsed

- 1/2 teaspoon freshly ground black pepper

- One large lemon, thinly sliced, seeds removed

- 1 1/2 teaspoons kosher salt

Preparation:

1. Preheat oven to 425 °F. In a baking dish, toss capers, beans & distribute them on the tray.

2. Spread mustard in beans & capers on the skin of every chicken. Put lemon pieces all around & beneath chicken & add insufficient water. Spice the dish with black pepper & sea salt & spray chicken with oil.

3. Insert the instant-read thermometer in chicken and roast it until skin becomes brown for thirty-five minutes

4. Switch the pan on the lower rack of the oven if the chicken starts to smoke while finishing the frying process.

5. Place prepared chicken in a bowl and decorate it with slices of lemon, capers, & beans. Put chicken sauce across the bowl and sprinkle it with parsley.

South-Western Chicken Salad

Prep Time: 10 min

Cook Time: 0 min

Serve: 6

Ingredients:

- 1 cup crushed tortilla chips

- 1 and 1/2 cups black beans

- 1 and 1/2 cups corn

- One avocado, diced

- One teaspoon minced garlic

- 1/2 cup plain Greek yogurt (use nonfat)

- 1/2 jalapeño, finely diced

- 1/2 red onion, diced

- Two teaspoons apple cider vinegar

- Two heaping teaspoons taco seasoning (use mild)

- Two teaspoons honey

- Two tomatoes, diced

- 3 Tablespoons extra virgin olive oil

- 3/4 cup shredded cheddar cheese

- 6 cups chopped romaine lettuce

- 6 cups cubed cooked chicken*

Dressing:

- handful chopped cilantro

- juice of 1 lime

- salt, to taste and if needed

Preparation:

Add all the ingredients to the bowl and mix them except salt Pour the dressing over the salad and toss it. Serve it cold.

The best turkey chili ever

Prep Time: 15 min

Cook Time: 60 min

Serve: 1

Ingredients:

- Three cloves of garlic, minced

- Two teaspoons hot sauce

- Two tablespoons olive oil

- Two tablespoons chili powder

- 2 pounds lean ground turkey

- 2 cups chicken or vegetable broth

- 1/2 teaspoon cayenne pepper (optional)

- One yellow pepper, chopped

- One yellow bell pepper, chopped

- One teaspoon garlic powder

- One teaspoon dried oregano

- One teaspoon dried basil

- One tablespoon brown sugar

- One sweet onion, finely chopped

- One red bell pepper, chopped

- 1/2 teaspoon sea salt

- 28oz crushed tomatoes

- 28oz black beans, drained

- 15oz petite diced tomatoes

- 15oz of kidney or pinto beans

Toppings: Sour cream, green onions, limes, shredded cheddar cheese

Preparation:

1. Heat the olive oil in a heavy bottom pot over medium-high & heat it till it shimmers. Add-In the ground turkey & simmer for 9 minutes, smashing it individually with a wooden spoon's help until it turned brown.

2. Add more olive oil if needed & whisk in onions & garlic.

3. Cook for 3 minutes before soften & fragrant.

4. Add peppers & again cook for three more minutes. Place the fried turkey in the pot again & then add the remaining ingredients to it. Stir & bring to a boil once combined.

5. Simmer this till the chili cooked completely 7 left it uncovered for 45 to 65 minutes until it becomes dense.

Warm Chicken Pasta Salad

Prep Time: 5 min

Cook Time: 18 min

Serve: 3

Ingredients:

- 375g dried rigatoni pasta

- 500g Lilydale Free Range Chicken Breast, trimmed

- One medium brown onion, thinly sliced

- One garlic clove, crushed

- 200g semi-dried tomatoes, drained, chopped

- 300ml pure cream

- 50g baby rocket

- 1/2 teaspoon dried chili flakes

- 1/4 cup olive oil

Preparation:

1. Take frypan and cook pasta until it becomes soft to follow the pasta packet's instructions and drain the remaining water. Along with that, heat 1 tbsp. Oil in a pan and add chicken to it.

2. Cook every side until it is completely cooked. Remove frypan from the stove, cover it & set it aside for 6 minutes. Take the remaining oil in a frypan, heat it over medium heat, and then add the onion. Cook for 4 to 6 minutes, mix frequently, or till the onion has softened. Onions, Garlic, & chili are added. Cook for 1 minute or till the smell is floral.

3. Now add cream, then cook for 4 to 6 minutes, or till the mixture thickens, stirring regularly.

4. Put a bowl of spaghetti, chicken, and rocket. Add the onions mixture. To combine, toss. Just serve.

Cinnamon Buckwheat Bowls

Prep Time: 5 min

Cook Time: 15 min

Serve: 1

Ingredients:

- ½ cup buckwheat groats, rinsed
- ½ cup almond milk or milk of choice
- ½ teaspoon cinnamon
- ½ cup water
- ½ teaspoon vanilla
- Honey to serve
- Sliced fruit to serve

Preparation:

1. In a small saucepan, add washed buckwheat grains, water, almond milk, cinnamon, and vanilla. Boil and then

simmer and cover with a lid. Cook over low heat for 10 minutes.

2. Turn off the heat and steam, covered, for an additional 5 minutes.

3. Pour with a fork and divide it into a bowl. Fill with fruit slices, sprinkle more milk and chopped honey if desired.

Salmon Salad

Prep Time: 10 min

Cook Time: 0 min

Serve: 1

Ingredients:

- 1 cup rocket

- oz. chicory leaves

- 1 tablespoon capers

- oz. avocado, peeled, stoned and sliced

- oz. smoked salmon slices

- 1/8 cup walnuts, chopped

- 1 large medjool date, pitted and chopped

- Juice of ¼ lemon

- 1 tablespoon extra-virgin olive oil

- 3/8 cup parsley, chopped

- ½ oz. celery leaves

- ¼ cup red onion, sliced

Preparation:

1. Place the salad leaves in a big bowl.

2. Mix all the other ingredients and serve on the leaves.

Arugula, Egg, and Charred Asparagus Salad

Prep Time: 5 min

Cook Time: 15 min

Serve: 4

Ingredients:

- oz. medium asparagus, trimmed
- ½ teaspoon black pepper, divided large eggs in shells
- 1 tablespoon fresh lemon juice
- oz. baby arugula
- 1 tablespoon extra-virgin olive oil
- 1 tablespoon water
- ¼ cup plain whole-milk Greek yogurt
- 1 teaspoon kosher salt, divided

Preparation:

1. Preheat broiler to high. Bring a small saucepan filled with water to a boil. Carefully add eggs. Cook for 8 minutes. Place eggs in a bowl filled with ice water and let stand for 2 minutes. Peel eggs, cut into quarters and sprinkle with ¼ teaspoon salt and 1/8 teaspoon pepper.

2. Combine olive oil, ¼ teaspoon salt, ¼ teaspoon pepper, and asparagus on a baking sheet. Spread in a single layer in pan. Boil for 3 minutes or until lightly charred. Remove asparagus mixture from the pan and cut into 2 inch pieces.

3. Combine remaining ¼ teaspoon salt, remaining 1/8 teaspoon pepper, yogurt, juice, and 1 tablespoon water in a medium bowl, stirring with a whisk. Add arugula and toss.

4. Arrange arugula mixture on a platter. Top with asparagus mixture and eggs. Enjoy!

Spring Vegetable and Quinoa Salad with Bacon

Prep Time: 5 min

Cook Time: 10 min

Serve: 4

Ingredients:

- 1 ¾ cups ginger-coconut quinoa
- cups fresh asparagus, cut diagonally into 1 inch pieces
- center-cut bacon slices, chopped
- 1 tablespoon unsalted butter
- tablespoons cider vinegar
- ½ cup frozen green peas
- teaspoons whole-grain
- Dijon mustard oz. baby spinach
- tablespoons sliced almonds, toasted

- 1 teaspoon black pepper

- 1 tablespoon fresh thyme leaves

- 1 tablespoon chopped fresh tarragon

- ½ cup chopped fresh flat-leaf parsley

Preparation:

1. Boil a large pot filled with water. Add asparagus and peas. Boil for 2 minutes, then drain. Plunge into a bowl of ice water and drain.

2. Cook the bacon in a large saucepan over medium-high heat, stirring occasionally. Remove bacon from the pan with a slotted spoon. Set aside.

3. Add vinegar, butter, and Dijon mustard to drippings in the pan, stirring with a whisk until butter melts. Add quinoa and pepper to the pan—cook for 1 minute.

4. Place quinoa mixture in a medium bowl. Add asparagus mixture, parsley, tarragon, thyme, and spinach, tossing to combine. Divide quinoa mixture among 4 plates; sprinkle evenly with reserved bacon and almonds.

Golden Chicory in Prosciutto Wraps

Prep Time: 20 min

Cook Time: 55 min

Serve: 1

Ingredients:

- heads of chicory

- slices prosciutto or Serrano ham

- 75 ml vegetable stock or white wine

- tablespoons butter

- tablespoons Dijon mustard

- ¼ cup whipping cream thyme sprigs

- slices, about 2 oz. melting cheese (cheddar is great)

- Sauté potatoes and green salad to serve

Preparation:

1. Preheat oven to 350 °F. Cut a cross from the base in the middle of the end of each chicory head. Fill the butter in the grooves, and then place the slices of Serrano ham in pairs on the work surface, overlapping them slightly. Paint the ham with mustard and spread the radish on top.

2. Pull each radish head away from you, comfortably wrapping it in the ham. Place the radish wrapped in an oven or small skillet, pour over the vegetable stock or white wine on top with the thyme sprigs. Cover the plate with loose foil and bake for 30-40 minutes until the radish is soft.

3. Unlock the plate, place the cheese slices on the chicory and bake, keep uncovered for another 6-8 minutes, until the cheese is melted and browned.

4. The radish is now ready to serve. For an extra touch, remove the chicory, place the pan on medium heat and boil

the juices with the cream for 4-5 minutes until they are rich and syrupy. Pour the sauce over the radish. Serve with sautéed potatoes and salad.

Vegetable Cabbage Soup

Prep Time: 5 min

Cook Time: 15 min

Serve: 6

Ingredients:

- ½ large head cabbage, chopped

- 1 large onion, chopped

- stalks celery, minced carrots, chopped

- tablespoons extra virgin olive oil cloves

- garlic, minced

- ½ teaspoon chili powder

- 1 can white beans, draineed and rinsed

- 1 can chopped fire-roasted tomatoes

- 1 pinch red pepper flakes

- 1 teaspoon thyme leaves

- cups low-sodium vegetable broth

- tablespoons freshly of chopped parsley, and more for garnish

- Kosher salt

- Freshly ground black pepper cups water

Preparation:

1. In a large pot over medium heat, heat olive oil. Add onion, celery, and carrots, and season with salt, pepper, and chili powder. Cook, stirring often, until vegetables are soft, 5 to 6 minutes. Stir in beans, thyme, and garlic and cook until garlic is fragrant, about 30 seconds.

2. Add broth and water, and bring to a simmer.

3. Stir in tomatoes and cabbage and simmer until cabbage is wilted, about 6 minutes. Remove from heat and stir in red pepper flakes, and parsley. Season to taste with salt and pepper. Garnish with more parsley, if desired. Enjoy!

Fresh Herb Frittata

Prep Time: 10 min

Cook Time: 15 min

Serve: 6

Ingredients:

- fresh eggs
- tablespoons chopped fresh parsley
- tablespoons chopped fresh oregano
- scallions, sliced thin, using both white and green parts
- ½ cup heavy cream
- ¾ cup finely grated parmesan cheese, divided into ½ cup and 1/4 cup portions
- Salt and pepper to taste

Preparation:

1. Preheat oven to 400 °F. In a medium mixing bowl, combine eggs, parsley, scallions, oregano, ½ cup of cheese, and heavy cream. Whisk together until thoroughly combined—season with salt and pepper, to taste.

2. In a 10-inch spicy cast iron pot, heat about 1 tablespoon of olive oil over medium heat. Add the egg mixture and cook for about 5 minutes or until the edges start to come out.

3. Sprinkle the remaining cup of cheese over the eggs.

4. Transfer the skillet to the oven and bake for 10-12 minutes, or until the cakes are puffy, the edges are visible and shake a little in the center.

5. Bake on low for about 30-45 seconds to brown the lid.

Herb-Roasted Olives and Tomatoes

Prep Time: 10 min

Cook Time: 20 min

Serve: 4

Ingredients:

- 1 cup Greek olives

- 1 cup garlic-stuffed olives

- cups cherry tomatoes

- 1 cup pitted ripe olives

- 1 tablespoon herbs de Provence

- tablespoons olive oil

- garlic cloves, peeled

- ¼ teaspoon pepper

Preparation:

1. Preheat oven to 425 °F. Combine cherry tomatoes, garlic-stuffed olives,

2. Greek olives, pitted ripe olives, and garlic cloves on a greased baking pan. Add oil and seasonings.

3. Toss to coat. Roast until tomatoes are softened, 15-20 minutes, stirring occasionally.

Grilled Asparagus with Caper Vinaigrette

Prep Time: 5 min

Cook Time: 10 min

Serve: 6

Ingredients:

- 1 ½ pounds asparagus spears, trimmed

- teaspoons caper, coarsely chopped

- 1 tablespoon red wine vinegar

- 1 garlic clove, minced

- tablespoons extra virgin olive oil

- ¼ cup small basil leaves

- ½ teaspoon Dijon mustard

- Cooking spray

- ½ teaspoon kosher salt, divided

- ¼ teaspoon freshly ground black pepper

Preparation:

1. Preheat grill to medium-high heat.

2. Place asparagus in a shallow dish. Add 1 tablespoon oil and ¼ teaspoon salt, tossing well to coat. Place asparagus on grill rack coated with cooking spray. Grill 4 minutes or until crisp-tender, turning after 2 minutes.

3. Combine remaining ¼ teaspoon salt, vinegar, mustard, and garlic. Stir with a whisk. Slowly pour remaining 2 tablespoons oil into vinegar mixture, stirring constantly with a whisk. Stir in capers. Arrange asparagus on a serving platter. Drizzle with vinaigrette, and sprinkle with basil.

Herby Pork with Apple & Chicory Salad

Prep Time: 5 min

Cook Time: 15 min

Serve: 4

Ingredients:

- oz. pork tenderloin, trimmed of any sinew and fat large apples, cored and sliced
- 270g pack chicory, leaves separated
- 1 tablespoon honey
- 1 tablespoon walnut oil
- 1 tablespoon chopped parsley
- 1 tablespoon chopped tarragon
- teaspoons wholegrain mustard
- Juice of 1 lemon

Preparation:

1. Preheat oven to 350°F. Grate pork with 1 teaspoon oil, 1 teaspoon mustard, and a few spices. Brown, transfer to a baking sheet and squeeze half of the herbs. Bake for 15 minutes until well cooked.

2. To make the salad, mix the lemon juice, honey, and the rest of the walnut oil and mustard. Period and add apples, radishes, and other herbs. Serve the sliced pork with the salad on the side.

Tomato Green Bean Soup

Prep Time: 15 min

Cook Time: 30 min

Serve: 4

Ingredients:

- 1 ½ cups diced fresh tomatoes

- ½ cup chopped onion

- ½ pound fresh green beans cut into 1 inch pieces

- ½ cup chopped carrots

- 1/8 cup minced fresh basil

- ½ garlic clove, minced

- ¼ teaspoon salt

- 1/8 teaspoon pepper

- 1 teaspoon butter

- cups reduced-sodium vegetable broth

Preparation:

1. In a large saucepan, sauté onion and carrots in butter for 5 minutes. Stir in the broth, green beans and garlic. Bring to a boil. Reduce heat. Cover and simmer until vegetables are tender.

2. Stir in the tomatoes, basil, salt and pepper. Cover and simmer 5 minutes longer.

www.ingramcontent.com/pod-product-compliance
Lightning Source LLC
Chambersburg PA
CBHW050752030426
42336CB00012B/1773